MARLEE & WE

Lessons from my Gut Health Disaster

Mastering Digestive Wellness

She had the foresight to strategize around driving change, but also the fortitude and patience to make that change happen, one small victory at a time.

BARB LOWMAN

Contents

1

Introduction

Hi, I'm Marlee! I'm a chronic digestive disease warrior, suffering from Crohn's Disease, IBS, SIBO, and severe autoimmune responses due to inflammation in my gut and whole body. It took years for my physicians to officially diagnose me, and I was officially diagnosed at the age of 18.

In November of 2022, I started having major symptoms that I thought was another Crohn's Disease flare. Through various doctor appointments, another colonoscopy, and 2 separate ER and Inpatient visits, I learned that nothing was physically wrong inside my body, other than the inflammation markers discovered in my blood.

I suffered so severely with diarrhea, cramping, and severe pain (10/10), that I had to wear diapers daily as I wasn't able to control my bowels. Not only that, but I went through a long period where I couldn't eat solid food by mouth for a few weeks. I put myself on a liquid-only diet, consisting of protein shakes and Gatorade/Pedialyte. After my liquid diet phase, I switched to eating mostly oatmeal for nutrition for another couple of weeks.

After the medication and diet still weren't working to heal my overall inflammation, I did some research and found the Low FODMAP diet. I asked my doctors if the Low FODMAP diet would be a good next step, and they agreed. I charged forward and did a ton of research on this diet, threw away foods that were potential triggers and worked with my partner to completely change the way we were eating and living.

After months of spending a lot of time, money, and effort on the Low FODMAP diet, I found a new way to manage my digestive and inflammatory symptoms through the gut-brain connection and mindfulness.

In my book, I hope to encourage all people who are struggling with their gut health, to find some answers to what might be triggering their symptoms, and find solace as you read my story, with science-backed strategies, and physician-approved tips on how to heal your gut health from the inside out.

2

Chapter 1: The Gut-Health Revolution

Ever wondered what gut inflammation and Godzilla share in common? Well, Gundersen's registered dietitian, Chris Swan, is here to break it down.

Think about it this way: Imagine inflammation as the wild chaos caused by the legendary movie monster, Godzilla. Just like how Godzilla rampages through cities catching everyone off guard, chronic inflammation does a similar thing inside our bodies. Over time, it paves the way for serious issues like chronic digestive diseases, heart disease, diabetes, arthritis, Alzheimer's, and autoimmune disorders – you know, the whole shebang.

Just as we'd want to rein in Godzilla's chaos, the same goes for inflammation. But the million-dollar question is: How can we actually do it?

The Gut Microbiome Unveiled & The Gut Ecosystem: An Overview

Imagine your gut as a bustling neighborhood packed with all sorts of tiny residents: bacteria, viruses, fungi, and other critters. Collectively, they make up what's called the "gut microbiome." Let's break down who's in the mix:

- **Bacteria:** These little guys are the VIPs of the gut. Some are like the friendly neighbors who help with chores (like digesting food), while others might cause a bit of trouble if they overstay their welcome.
- **Viruses:** Think of these as the tiny superheroes that focus on specific bacteria. They're like the pest control of the gut, keeping bacteria in check.
- **Fungi:** You've got some yeasts and molds hanging around too. They're not as numerous as bacteria, but they play a role in digestion and getting nutrients from your food.
- **Archaea:** These guys are the archaeologists of the bunch - ancient microorganisms with their own quirks.
- **Other Microorganisms:** And there's more! Single-celled creatures like eukaryotes join the party, adding to the diversity.

Remember, your gut microbiome is like a fingerprint—it's unique to you. And when it's diverse and balanced, it's like having a harmonious neighborhood that keeps your digestion, immune system, and even your mood in good shape.

Gut-Body Interactions

Picture this: your gut and brain are like the ultimate BFFs who are constantly chatting. They're not sending texts, but they're using something called the "gut-brain connection." This is the cool way they talk to each other.

So, you know when you get butterflies in your stomach before a big event? That's your gut and brain having a chit-chat. They're sharing all sorts of news, like how you're feeling, what you're eating, and even if there's any trouble going on down there.

But it's a two-way street. Your gut can also send signals to your brain. Like if you eat something funky, your gut might tell your brain, "Hey, something's not right here!" That's why sometimes your mood can be influenced by what's going on in your gut

Basically, your gut and brain are besties who never stop talking, and all this communication has a big impact on how you feel, think, and even how healthy you are. Let's dive into how this whole gut-brain chat affects things like your body's defense team (that's your immune system) and those pesky red flags (inflammation).

So, when your gut and brain are chitchatting, they're also giving a heads-up to your immune system. Imagine your immune system as those superhero guards at the gate. When your gut signals something's not right (like bad food or invaders), the guards gear up to fight off the bad guys. This is why a happy gut can lead to a strong immune system that's ready to tackle anything.

But here's the twist: sometimes, when the gut-brain chat goes off track, it can create confusion. Imagine the guards getting a false alarm and rushing around for no reason. This can lead to chronic inflammation – like a never-ending fire drill. Chronic inflammation is like a sneaky villain that can mess with your health, causing all sorts of problems from allergies to serious diseases.

So, bottom line: when your gut and brain have a clear, smooth convo, your immune system stays in superhero mode and inflammation behaves. But when their chat gets haywire, it's like a comic book chaos, and that's when immunity and inflammation get all tangled up.

Factors Influencing the Gut

Picture your gut as a super sensitive control center that's influenced by everything you do, eat, and even where you hang out. Yep, diet, lifestyle, and your surroundings can totally shake things up in there.

- **Diet:** What you put in your mouth matters big time. Think of it as fuel for your gut's engine. If you're feeding it junk food all the time, it's like running your car on dirty gas. But when you give it good stuff - lots of veggies, fiber, and nutrients - it's like treating your gut to premium fuel. And that helps the good gut buddies thrive while keeping the troublemakers at bay.
- **Lifestyle:** Your day-to-day routine can flip switches in your gut. Stress? Yeah, it's like hitting a panic button. Your gut's like, "Whoa, what's happening?!" Regular exercise? That's like giving your gut a high-five. It loves movement. Plus, sleep is like a spa day for your gut - when you snooze, it gets to work on repairs and maintenance.
- **Environment:** Where you live and what you're exposed to matters too. Air pollution, chemicals, and even the germs around you can mess with your gut buddies. A clean, green environment is like a cozy home for them to hang out, while a polluted one is like trying to have a party in a trash heap.

Long story short, your gut's like a sponge, soaking up everything from your choices to your surroundings. Feed it good, treat it well, and your gut will be your biggest cheerleader.

Alright, let's talk about how your brain's mood swings can mess with your gut vibes. Imagine your gut as this sensitive friend who's super connected to your emotions. When you're feeling all happy and chill, your gut's like, "Cool, we're good to go!" But when stress or anxiety hits, it's like your gut starts to stress too. It's like they're on a walkie-talkie, sharing all the feels.

Here's the twist: Your gut has its own little gang called the "gut microbiome." They're like the sidekicks in this story. When your mood takes a nosedive, these little sidekicks might act up, causing tummy troubles. It's like they're throwing a tantrum because you're not feeling great.

And guess what? This whole mood-gut thing is a two-way street. When your gut buddies are happy and thriving, they can send signals back to your brain, giving you a mood boost. So it's like a loop of emotions and gut reactions.

In short, your mental health is like the DJ of this gut party. When the music's good, your gut dances along. When it's off, well, things can get a bit awkward on the dance floor. So, keep your vibes positive, and your gut will be singing along happily.

3

Chapter 2: Gut Health's Impact on Wellness

Digestion and Nutrient Absorption

Friends, it's time to get down to business with your gut's ultimate food-breaking party! Imagine your gut as a wild concert where the main act is breaking down your food into smaller pieces. Let's break it down even more:

When you munch on that burger or chomp on those veggies, your gut's like a superstar band with special instruments. These instruments are enzymes, and they're like the rockstars that break down your food into its tiniest parts. It's like turning a huge sandwich into bite-sized pieces that your body can actually use.

And guess what? There's a super smart article that dives deep into this food party. Check out "The Role of Enzyme Supplementation in Digestive Disorders" by Roxas M. (2008) in the Alternative Medicine Review. It's like the backstage pass to understanding how these enzymes work their magic. It's all about how these enzymes help your body absorb the good stuff from your food and make sure nothing goes to waste.

So, your gut's not just a foodie – it's a food magician too, turning your eats into the fuel your body needs. Rock on, gut, rock on!

Alright, listen up! Nutrient absorption is like your body's treasure hunt for all the good stuff in your food. Imagine your gut as a treasure chest and your bloodstream as the explorer. So, after your gut breaks down food into its tiny pieces, your body gets to work. It grabs those nutrients - like vitamins, minerals, and other goodies - and sends them on a journey through your bloodstream.

Nutrient absorption is like getting your body's VIP pass to all the essential nutrients it needs to function at its best. And here's why this treasure hunt is a big deal: all those nutrients are like little helpers that keep your body running smoothly. They're the energy boosters, the brain-boosting agents, and the defenders against all sorts of health issues. So, next time you eat, know that your body's on a mission to snatch up those nutrients and make you feel awesome!

Mental Health and Mood

Friends, let's dive into some brainy business! Picture in your mind that your gut and brain are BFFs who are on speed dial. This hotline they use to chat is called the "gut-brain axis." It's like your own private phone line connecting your belly and your brain.

But here's the cool twist: They're not just texting emojis to each other. They're using special messengers called neurotransmitters. Think of these guys as tiny delivery people, zipping back and forth between your gut and brain, carrying messages like "Hey, we're stressed!" or "Time to chill!"

Want to geek out on this? Check out "The gut-brain axis: Interactions between enteric microbiota, central and enteric nervous systems" by Marilia Carabotti (2015) in the Annals of Gastroenterology. It's like the backstage pass to understanding how these messengers work their magic. So, your gut-brain axis is like the ultimate gossip line, where messages fly and emotions flow. It's a crazy cool way your belly and brain team up to keep you feeling good.

Let's have a deeper heart-to-heart about something important: the secret connection between your gut and your mood. You know those days when your tummy feels off and suddenly your mood takes a nosedive? Well, it's not just in your head – it's in your gut too.

Imagine your gut as a second brain, like a mood-sensing sidekick. It's got this whole crew of bacteria, and they're like your gut's little therapists. They send signals to your real brain, and those signals can actually affect how you feel.

This quote from psychologist Dr. Kimberley Wilson sums it up perfectly: "Stress and nutrition are a two-way street. Stress can influence food choices, and what you eat affects how well your brain and body handle stress." What we eat affects how we feel, and how we feel can influence our digestion. So, if your gut buddies aren't happy, they might mess with your mood.

But here's the silver lining: When you treat your gut right, it's like sending love notes to your mood. Healthy foods, stress relief, and self-care – they're all part of the self-love package for your gut and mind. So remember, taking care of your belly is like giving your mood a warm hug.

Immune System Support

Remember the Godzilla analogy? Your gut is like the ultimate defender of your body, and it's got a secret weapon: your immune response. Think of it as your gut's personal superhero team that's always on standby.

Here's the deal: Your gut buddies play a huge role in training your immune system. They're like the coaches, teaching your immune cells to recognize the good guys from the bad guys. And when those bad guys try to sneak in, your immune system goes all ninja on them.

But wait, there's more! Your gut also knows how to prevent friendly fire. Autoimmune reactions happen when your immune system goes a little haywire and starts attacking your own cells. But with a well-balanced gut, those friendly-fire episodes are way less likely. It's like having a superhero team that's super-focused and doesn't accidentally beat up the good guys.

So, bottom line: treat your gut well, and it'll keep your immune system in superhero mode, ready to protect you from all sorts of trouble.

4

Chapter 3: Setting the Stage for Mastery

Reflecting on Personal Gut Health Disasters

Friends, I encourage you all to assess your gut health and other autoimmune challenges, stay tuned until the end when I'll help lay out an assessment for you! As a chronic gut warrior myself (sidenote: we're all warriors!) I know firsthand how challenging it can be to be in another storm of digestive distress. I've had more than I can keep track of and have been everywhere from small clinics to Mayo Clinic multiple times trying to get the right answers to my health and heal my body holistically.

I wasn't able to heal my body holistically until I took a deeper picture of my body and health as a whole, utilizing both science-backed strategies, and recommendations from my healthcare team, and taking a deep dive into other methods myself. I encourage all of you to find out what works best for YOU and to be your own advocate as you continue to work further with your health system team.

Embracing the Growth Mindset

Let's dive into a little mindset makeover! You know, life throws us all sorts of curveballs, especially when it comes to our health. But guess what? We've got the ultimate tool in our toolkit: a growth mindset.

Think of it as a pair of super cool glasses that change how you see things. Do you know those health challenges that might seem like huge mountains? Well, with a growth mindset, they're more like exciting adventures waiting to be conquered.

Imagine this: every bump in the road is a chance to learn, grow, and become even stronger. It's like turning setbacks into setups for success. Yeah, it's not always easy, but it's the secret sauce to flipping the script in those tough times.

So, get ready to strap on those growth mindset glasses and see a future that's full of possibilities. Challenges? Bring 'em on – you've got a whole new way to handle them now!

Navigating the Book's Journey

Throughout the rest of our journey together, I will provide you with an informal understanding of science-backed strategies and solutions to help heal your gut and helpful info on how you, too, can master your digestive wellness. My hope is that you are able to walk away feeling like you have practical tips that can not only improve your gut health but improve your overall wellness. Your livelihood is of top importance!

5

Chapter 4: Unveiling the Solutions

Diet and Nutrition Adjustments

Friends, you may remember in my introduction that one of the first methods I took to ease my digestive symptoms in my disaster was following the Low FODMAP diet, backed by Monash University. The low FODMAP diet is like a superhero diet for your gut! Imagine you have this secret team of foods that swoop in to save the day when your tummy's not feeling its best.

FODMAPs are like these tiny things in certain foods that can cause chaos in your gut. They stand for Fermentable Oligosaccharides, Disaccharides, Monosaccharides, and Polyols. Yeah, it sounds all sciencey, but basically, they're the troublemakers behind bloating, cramps, and other gut and autoimmune issues.

So, the low FODMAP diet is like calling in the reinforcements. You stick to foods that are low in these troublemakers and boom - your gut's happier. Some gut-friendly foods you can enjoy are strawberries, blueberries, carrots, rice, and chicken. These guys won't cause your gut to throw a tantrum.

But remember, it's like a temporary mission. Once your gut's feeling better, you can slowly bring back other foods and see how your tummy reacts. It's all about finding what makes your gut do a happy dance!

So, if your gut's been giving you a hard time, the low FODMAP diet might just be the hero it needs. Time to rescue your tummy and live that gut-friendly life, but no worries, you won't have to live on such a limited diet forever!

Let's break it down into some simple gut-friendly guidelines!

- **Fiber is Your Friend:** Load up on fiber-rich foods like fruits, veggies, whole grains, and legumes. Fiber is like a broom that sweeps your gut clean and keeps things moving smoothly.
- **Probiotics Power:** Bring in the probiotics! These are like the good gut buddies that help balance things out. You'll find them in yogurt, kefir, sauerkraut, and other fermented foods.
- **Hydrate, Hydrate, Hydrate:** Drink plenty of water. Your gut needs it to work its magic, from digestion to absorption.
- **Diversify Your Plate:** Mix up your meals with a variety of foods. Each type brings its own set of nutrients to the gut party.
- **Cut Back on Processed Stuff:** Processed foods with added sugars and unhealthy fats can mess with your gut. Opt for real, whole foods as much as possible.
- **Moderation is Key:** Enjoy treats in moderation. A little indulgence won't hurt, but make sure your everyday choices support gut health.
- **Chew, Chew, Chew:** Take your time while eating. Chewing well helps your gut handle the digestion process more smoothly.
- **Manage Stress:** Stress is like the party pooper for your gut. Try

relaxation techniques like deep breathing, meditation, or yoga to keep stress in check.

- **Regular Mealtimes:** Stick to regular eating times. Your gut loves routine, and it helps keep everything balanced.
- **Listen to Your Body:** Pay attention to how your gut reacts to different foods. If something doesn't agree with you, give it a break.

Remember, it's all about treating your gut like the VIP it is. So, load up on the good stuff, keep things balanced, and your gut will be the happiest camper in town!

Lifestyle Modifications

Let's talk about the three amigos that can seriously boost your gut game: exercise, stress management, and sleep. These aren't just random things you do – they're like the secret sauce for a happy gut!

- **Exercise:** Think of exercise as your gut's daily workout. When you get moving, you're not only keeping your body fit, but you're also giving your gut some love. Exercise can help keep your digestion smooth by preventing things from getting all sluggish. Plus, it's like a mood booster for both your brain and your gut buddies. They all love a good sweat session!
- **Stress Management:** Ah, stress – the gut's arch-nemesis. When you're all stressed out, your gut buddies can feel it too. But here's the kicker: When you manage stress, you're handing your gut a bouquet of roses. Techniques like deep breathing, meditation, or even a simple walk in the park can calm your gut and keep it from acting up.
- **Sleep:** Imagine sleep as a spa day for your gut. When you catch those Z's, your gut gets to work repairing and rejuvenating itself.

It's like the ultimate "me time" for your belly. On the flip side, when you don't get enough sleep, it's like leaving your gut buddies with a cranky babysitter – things can get messy.

So, remember, it's not just about what you eat, but how you live. These lifestyle buddies – exercise, stress management, and sleep – they're like the entourage that keeps your gut feeling fantastic. Give them some love, and your gut will thank you with a happy dance!

Practical Tips and Hacks

Alright, time for some gut-friendly hacks that are as easy as pie if you need immediate relief! These quick tips are like little boosts for your gut health:

- **Stay Hydrated:** Sip on water throughout the day. Hydration keeps your gut working smoothly.
- **Add Fiber:** Sneak in fiber-rich foods like veggies and fruits. They're like gut superheroes.
- **Eat Probiotics:** If you can tolerate lactose, yogurt, kefir, and fermented foods are like friendly gut helpers. They balance things out. If you're allergic to lactose or find out through the Low FODMAP diet that lactose is one of your current triggers, I recommend taking a pre and probiotic supplement. (sidenote - this is a recommendation from my holistic health/integrated wellness physician)
- **Limit Sugar:** Cut back on added sugars. Too much sugar can mess with your gut buddies.
- **Mindful Eating:** Pay attention while you eat. It helps your gut digest food more effectively.
- **Get Moving:** Even a short walk after meals can help your gut digest

better.

- **De-stress:** Find stress-busters that work for you. It's like giving your gut a spa day.
- **Sleep Well:** Aim for 7-9 hours of quality sleep. Your gut loves a good night's rest.
- Limit Processed Foods: Minimize foods with additives and artificial stuff. Your gut prefers real food.

Incorporate these hacks into your daily routine to build gut-friendly habits:

- **Meal Prep:** Plan meals with gut-friendly foods, and prep them in advance for a stress-free week.
- **Mindful Snacking:** Choose nuts, seeds, or veggies for quick and satisfying snacks.
- **Food Journaling:** Keep track of how different foods make you feel. It's like your gut's diary.
- **Herbal Teas:** Sip on ginger or peppermint tea. They're like soothing hugs for your gut.

Remember, these tips are like little puzzle pieces that create a big picture of a happy gut. You've got this – one small step at a time!

6

Chapter 5: Empowering Your Journey

Long-term Maintenance

Alright, let's talk long-term gut greatness! Making lasting improvements is like growing a garden - it takes time, care, and a sprinkle of patience. Here's how to nurture your gut for the long haul:

- **Consistency is Key:** Keep up those healthy habits. It's not about perfection but about making good choices most of the time.
- **Gradual Changes:** Don't go from zero to hero overnight. Slowly introduce healthier foods and habits to let your gut adjust.
- **Keep Learning:** Stay curious about gut health. The more you know, the better choices you'll make.
- **Listen to Signals:** Your gut's like a talkative friend. Pay attention to how it reacts to different foods and situations.
- **Stay Hydrated:** Drink water daily to keep things flowing smoothly in your gut.
- **Prioritize Sleep:** Aim for consistent, quality sleep. It's like charging your gut's batteries.

- **Manage Stress:** Find stress-relief strategies that work for you. A happy mind equals a happy gut.
- **Celebrate Progress:** Every small win counts. Celebrate each step you take toward a healthier gut.

Now, let's talk about building that tough gut ecosystem:

- **Diverse Diet:** Eat a wide variety of foods. A diverse diet supports a diverse gut microbiome.
- **Probiotics and Prebiotics:** Consume foods with probiotics (like yogurt) and prebiotics (like fiber-rich foods) to feed your gut buddies.
- **Limit Antibiotics:** Use antibiotics only when necessary. They can mess with your gut's delicate balance.
- **Moderate Alcohol:** Enjoy alcohol in moderation. Excessive drinking can harm your gut health.
- **Regular Check-ins:** Regularly assess your gut health. If things feel off, make tweaks to get back on track.
- **Stay Active:** Keep moving! Regular exercise is like a party your gut buddies love attending.
- **Laugh Often:** Seriously, laughter is good for your gut. It reduces stress and boosts mood.
- **Stay Positive:** A positive outlook can impact your gut health. Embrace challenges with a growth mindset.

Remember, building a resilient gut ecosystem is like constructing a solid foundation for a house. The stronger it is, the better it can weather storms. So, keep nurturing and supporting your gut - it's your ultimate health buddy for life!

Reader's Reflection and Action

In Chapter 3, I encouraged you to take an assessment of your gut health. Here's a guided self-assessment to check in with yourself! Grab a pen and paper, and write these down in a journal or another method that you prefer that you're able to go back and reflect on.

Step 1: Lifestyle Check

Take a look at your daily routine and habits:

- **Diet:** Write down what you typically eat in a day. Include foods rich in fiber, whole grains, veggies, and fruits.
- **Hydration:** Note how much water you drink daily. Are you staying well-hydrated?
- **Exercise:** Jot down your weekly exercise routine. Do you engage in regular physical activity?
- **Stress:** Reflect on how you manage stress. Are you using techniques like deep breathing or meditation?
- **Sleep:** Write down your nightly sleep duration. Are you getting 7-9 hours of quality sleep?

Step 2: Gut Signals

Pay attention to what your gut is telling you:

- **Digestion:** Do you experience bloating, gas, or discomfort after eating certain foods?
- **Regular Bowel Movements:** Are your bowel movements regular, and do they feel comfortable?
- **Energy Levels:** How's your energy throughout the day? Do you experience fatigue or crashes?
- **Mood:** Reflect on your mood. Are you feeling generally positive,

or do you often experience mood swings?

Step 3: Food and Mood Connection

Consider how your food choices impact your emotions:

- **Food-Mood Relationship:** Do you notice any connection between what you eat and how you feel emotionally?
- **Cravings:** Are you frequently craving sugary or processed foods?

Step 4: Growth Mindset and Stress

Assess your mindset and stress management:

- **Mindset:** Do you approach challenges with a growth mindset, seeing them as opportunities for learning?
- **Stress Management:** How do you manage stress? Are you practicing relaxation techniques?

Step 5: Action Plan

Based on your assessment, identify areas you'd like to improve:

- **Prioritize:** Choose one or two areas you want to work on, like adding more fiber to your diet or practicing stress-relief techniques.
- **Set Goals:** Set specific, achievable goals for each area. For example, aim to include a serving of probiotic-rich food each day.
- **Plan:** Create a plan to implement your goals. It could be meal prepping, scheduling exercise, or practicing mindfulness.
- **Monitor:** Keep track of your progress. Use a journal to note changes in digestion, mood, and energy levels.

- **Adjust:** Be flexible and adjust your plan as needed. Your gut's unique, so what works for someone else might need tweaking for YOU.

Remember, this assessment is like checking the roadmap to your gut health journey. It's all about learning, improving, and enjoying the process. You've got this!

Shifting the Mindset

Let's take a peek into the growth mindset once more and explore how it's the secret sauce for ongoing success in your gut health journey:

Step 1: Embrace the Learning Curve

- See every step as a learning opportunity. When you're trying new gut-friendly habits, whether it's adding more fiber or managing stress, know that it's okay to stumble. Each stumble is like a chance to learn what works best for you. It's not about being perfect from the get-go; it's about growing over time.

Step 2: Celebrate Progress

- Acknowledge your victories, big or small. Did you manage to add more veggies to your meals this week? Awesome! Give yourself a high-five. These wins are like little motivational boosts that keep you on track.

Step 3: Shift Focus from Setbacks

- Instead of seeing setbacks as failures, view them as valuable feedback. If you indulged in that slice of cake even though you planned to skip sugary treats, don't beat yourself up. Instead, understand what triggered the decision and how you can handle similar situations better in the future.

Step 4: Keep the Long-Term Picture in Mind

- Remember, gut health is a journey, not a destination. It's not about short-term fixes but creating lasting changes. Having a growth mindset means you're in it for the long haul. Visualize how your efforts today will contribute to your overall well-being down the road.

Step 5: Embrace Challenges

- Challenges are like the weights at the gym – they make you stronger. When you encounter a tough moment in your gut health journey, view it as a chance to flex your growth mindset muscles. How can you learn from this challenge? How can you pivot and keep moving forward?

Step 6: Use Self-Talk Wisely

- Your inner voice is like your biggest cheerleader (or critic). So, make sure it's cheering you on! When you catch yourself thinking negatively or feeling defeated, reframe those thoughts. Instead of "I can't do this," switch to "I'm learning and improving every day."

Step 7: Seek Inspiration

- Surround yourself with inspiration. Follow gut health success stories, read motivational books or articles, and connect with like-minded individuals who are also on a growth journey. Sharing experiences and insights can keep you motivated.

Remember, a growth mindset isn't just about your actions; it's about your attitude. It's the belief that you have the power to improve, learn, and adapt. So, keep that growth mindset front and center in your gut health adventure, and you'll be set for continued success!

7

Conclusion: The Road to Mastery

L et's wrap up this gut health transformational journey with some bite-size takeaways. My hope is that whoever reads this can take charge of their own health, find gut health relief, and continue to master your digestive wellness!

- **Gut Health is Vital:** Your gut health impacts your overall well-being – from digestion to immunity, mood, and more.
- **Growth Mindset is Key:** Embrace a growth mindset. See challenges as opportunities, celebrate progress, and keep learning.
- **Start Small:** Make gradual changes to your diet and lifestyle. It's not about perfection but progress.
- **Fiber and Probiotics:** Load up on fiber-rich foods and introduce probiotics to support your gut's good buddies.
- **Hydration and Movement:** Drink water, stay active, and keep your gut in motion for smoother digestion.
- **Stress Management:** Practice stress-relief techniques like deep breathing, meditation, and mindful living.
- **Mind-Body Connection:** Understand the link between your gut and mental health. A happy gut often means a happier you.

- **Celebrate Wins:** Acknowledge every achievement, no matter how small. They add up and keep you motivated.
- **Long-Term Perspective:** See your gut health journey as a marathon, not a sprint. It's about sustained well-being.
- **Embrace Setbacks:** Learn from setbacks; they're part of the process. Reframe them as opportunities to grow.
- **Transform Your Mindset:** Shift your self-talk from negativity to positivity. Believe in your ability to change and improve.
- **Connection and Support:** Surround yourself with inspiration and like-minded individuals who uplift your journey.

Remember, this isn't just about gut health; it's about your transformation from someone who faced gut health challenges to someone who's mastering it. Every step you take, every choice you make, contributes to your evolution. Keep that growth mindset shining bright as you embrace your own journey from "gut health disaster" to "gut health mastery." And always remember, food is your friend, not your enemy!

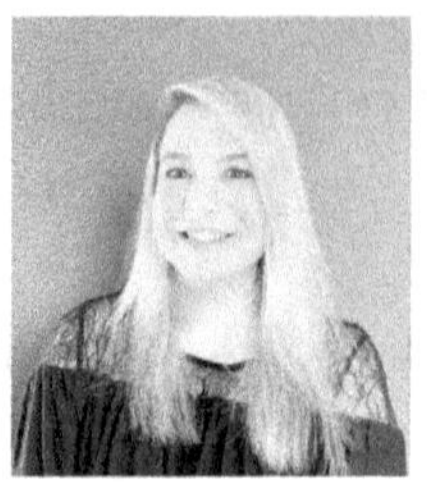

About the Author

Meet Marlee, a gutsy go-getter living life to the fullest in Madison, WI, alongside her boyfriend Brett. A true warrior, Marlee battles Crohn's Disease with unwavering strength, turning her challenges into triumphs.

With her tailored lifestyle adjustments, Marlee has conquered the art of savoring life's flavors and embracing newfound freedoms. When she's not curating her journey to wellness, you'll find her vibing to the beat of EDM music, crushing project management, exploring new horizons through travel, and relishing in the local culinary scene.

A devoted reader and writer, Marlee finds solace in the pages of books and crafts her own narratives under the pen name "Marlee & We."

With an insatiable passion for helping others, Marlee's mission is to share her wisdom and insights, guiding fellow travelers on their own paths to well-being. Get ready to join her on a journey that celebrates life, love, and the healing power of resilience.